T0022819

SLOW DOWN, TAKE A NAP

A CELEBRATION OF THE SIESTA

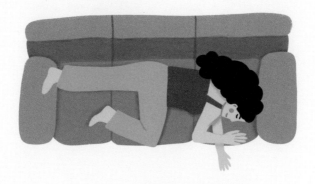

illustrated by MARINA OLIVEIRA

duopress

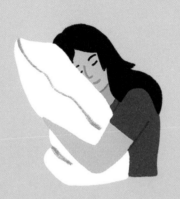

nap

noun

a sweet, short slumber that softly slips in between sunrise and sunset

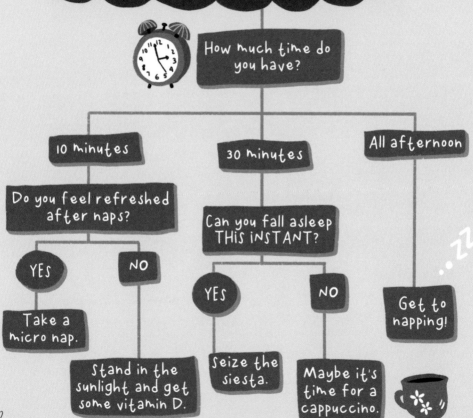

2

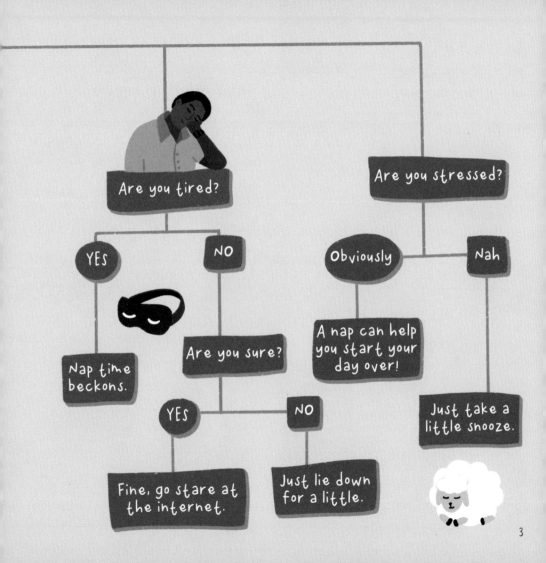

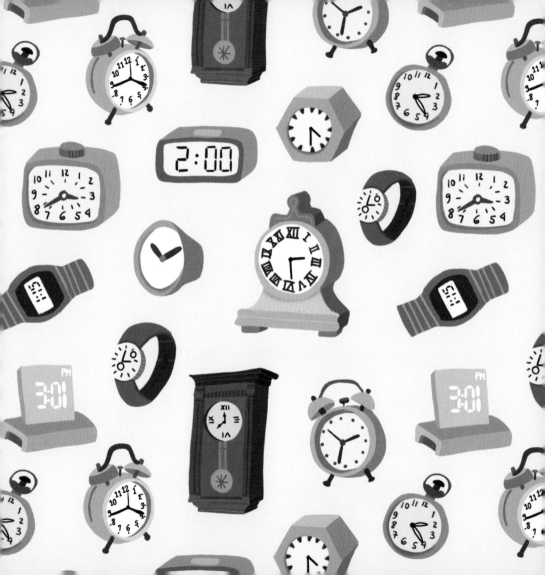

Nap time IS MY HAPPY HOUR

YOU ARE GETTING SLEEPY...

MAINTAIN A PERFECT SLEEPING CLIMATE

Sleep hygiene, or habits that prime you for sleep, will help you snooze at any time of day. Experts say a room temperature between 65 and 72 degrees Fahrenheit is ideal. Keep your socks on to warm your feet—toasty toes signal to your brain that it's time to snooze. Use blackout curtains to make the room dark. Diffuse the calming aroma of lavender essential oil. Consider a white noise machine to drown out city noise or loud thoughts.

READ A BOOK

In a randomized trial, people who read a book before trying to sleep experienced less sleep disturbance.

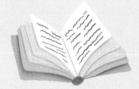

COUNT SHEEP—ACTUALLY, DON'T

Legend has it that sheepherders in medieval Britain had to count every member of their flock before going to sleep at night. It must have set their minds at ease to know all their charges were safe in the herd. Another ancient text references Islamic culture as the origin of counting sheep. In modern times, however, counting sheep has not held up well in research—a 2002 study found that it took longer for sleep-deprived sheep-counters to nod off than those who didn't use the technique.

VISUALIZE SERENITY

Picture a running waterfall or babbling brook. Imagine what it's like to be in a calm place, like on a beach — thinking of sights, smells, and feelings.

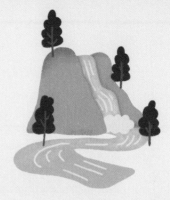

PLAN FOR POSTPRANDIAL DROWSINESS

A natural dip in wakefulness happens after lunch. Take advantage of this circadian fluctuation with food or drink containing tryptophan — an amino acid famous for making people sleepy — like turkey, cheese, oatmeal, tuna, or warm milk. Eating large meals also induces drowsiness, so go for the lunch buffet!

CENTER YOUR BODY AND MIND

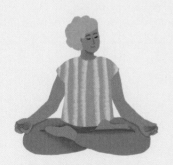

Breath work, such as box breathing (visualizing a square path as you breathe in and out, 4 seconds at a time) or the 4–7–8 method (inhale for 4 seconds, hold for 7, exhale for 8, repeat), can help you drift off. So can muscle relaxation exercises, where you tense and then relax one muscle at a time, starting at your toes and ending at your head. Or, try the Military Method, page 121.

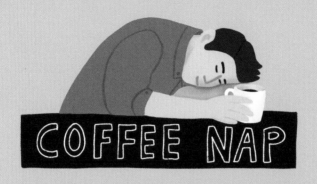

COFFEE NAP

a short daytime snooze taken immediately
after drinking a caffeinated beverage

a.k.a. stimulant nap, nappuccino

TIME: 20 to 30 minutes

Chugging coffee right before a nap might sound
counterproductive, but there is a method to this madness:
Caffeine takes effect about 30 minutes after it is ingested...
so if you drain a cup of coffee just before a 30-minute nap,
you will wake up feeling more alert and ready to face the day.

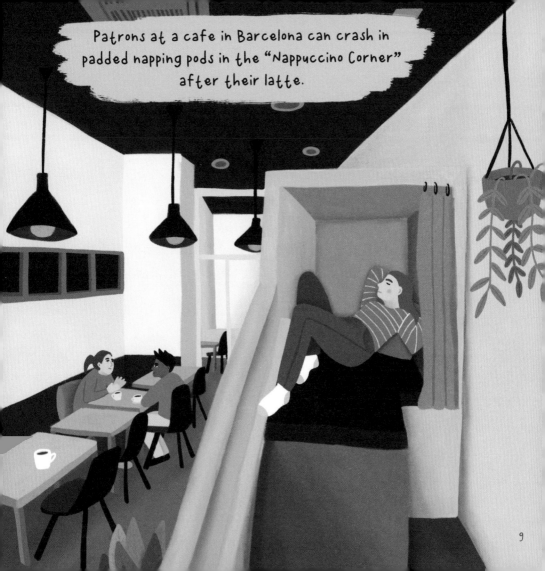

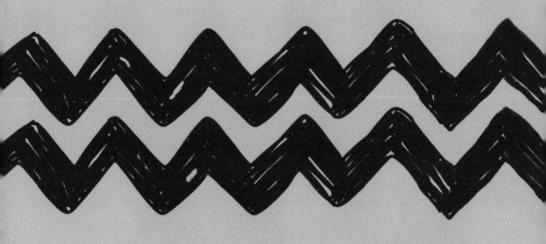

"LEARN FROM YESTERDAY, LIVE FOR TODAY, LOOK FOR TOMORROW, REST THIS AFTERNOON."

—Charles M. Schulz, *Peanuts* creator

11

What's Your Napping PERSONALITY?

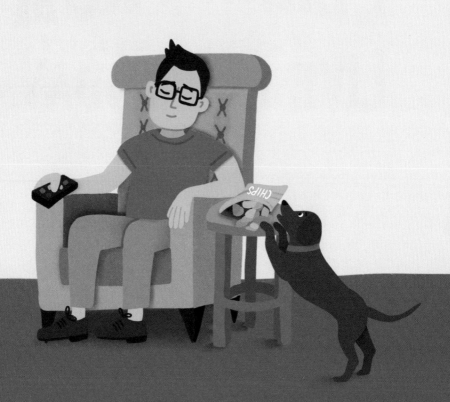

JUST RESTING MY EYES

Common among individuals who harbor a deep desire for sleep but are unable to achieve it during daylight hours. "Resting" may include a sleep mask, freshly sliced cucumbers, or a pillow secured on top of the eyelids to force them closed. Sleep is furtive, but desirable, for this individual. Proceed with caution, as the subject may be using a "nap" as a disguise for eavesdropping.

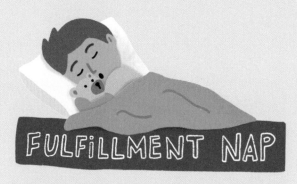

FULFiLLMENT NAP

daytime sleep needed to aid growth or
recovery, e.g., for a child or an athlete

TIME: 30 minutes or more

NAP WHEN THE KIDS NAP

From the moment they emerge as tiny snoozing machines, children rely on naps
for growth, learning, energy, and mood. (Hence why new parents often follow
the age-old advice about sleeping when the baby sleeps.)
The need for sleep doesn't stop at childhood—teenagers need more than adults
and are often overscheduled and dragged out of bed early for school.
They benefit from naps too!

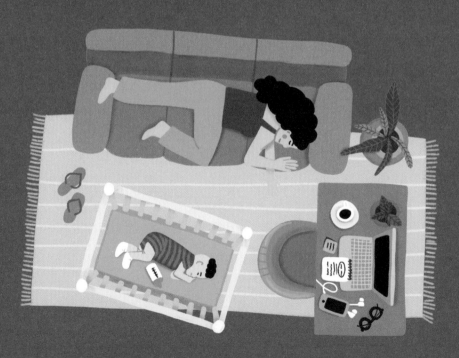

Little eyelids, cease your winking;
Little orbs, forget to beam;
Little soul, to slumber sinking,
Let the fairies rule your dream.
Breezes, through the lattice sweeping,
Sing their lullabies the while —
And a star-ray, softly creeping
To thy bedside, woos thy smile.
But no song nor ray entrancing
Can allure thee from the spell
Of the tiny fairies dancing
O'er the eyes they love so well.
See, we come in countless number —
I, their queen, and all my court —
Haste, my precious one, to slumber
Which invites our fairy sport.

—EUGENE FIELD, "AN INVITATION TO SLEEP"

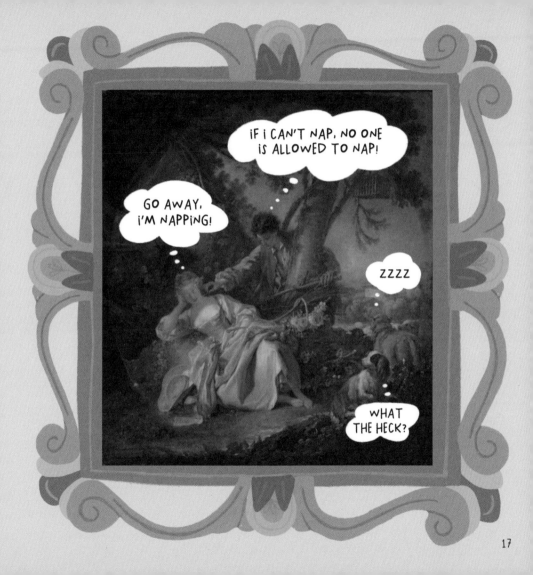

17

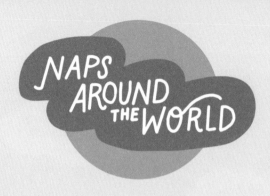

iNEMURI

The Japanese art of "sleeping while present"
— a.k.a. the sign of a hardworking employee.

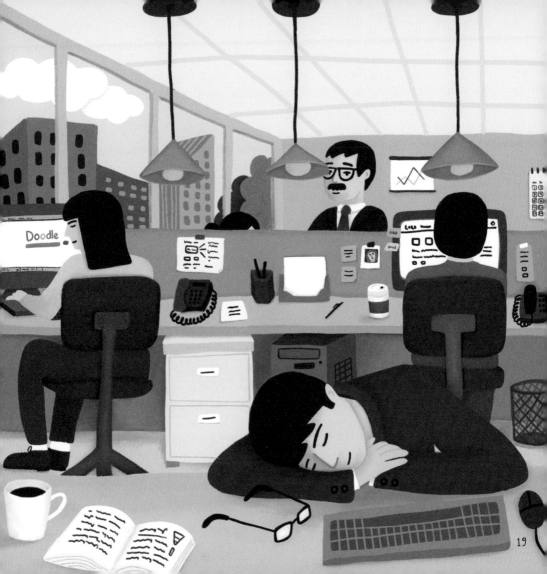

19

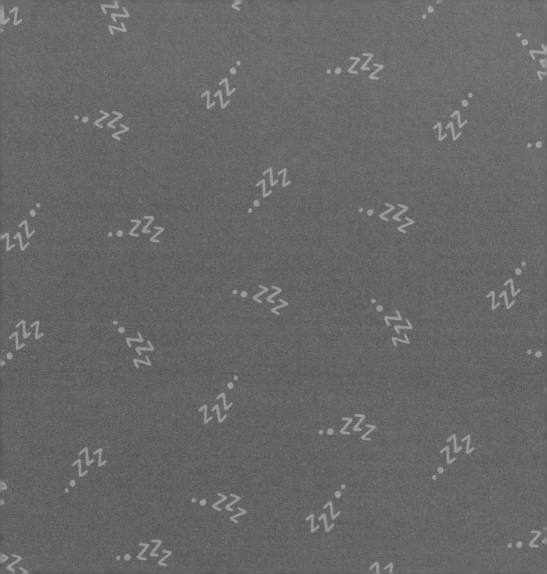

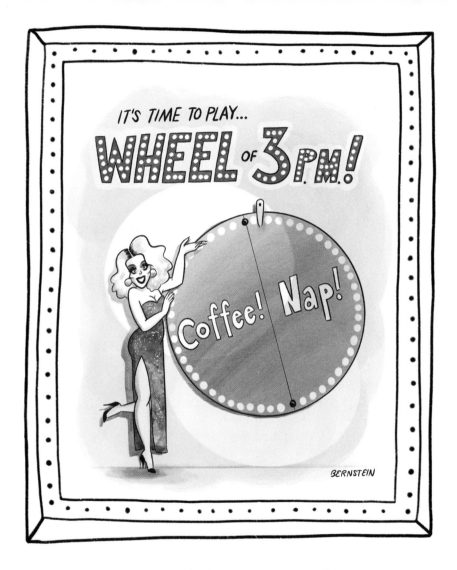

21

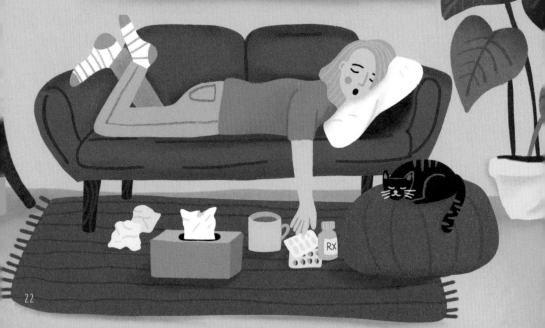

ESSENTIAL NAP

a nap taken to recover during an illness, to help your body fight infection and heal itself, and to boost the immune system

TIME: as long as needed

22

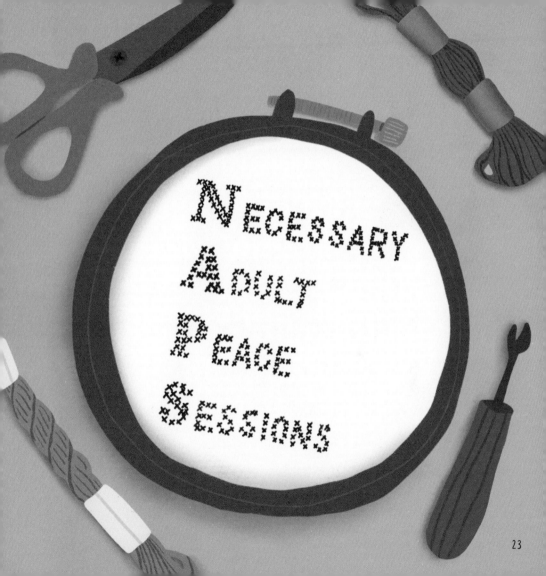

23

WHAT DOES YOUR SLEEPING MASK SAY ABOUT YOU?

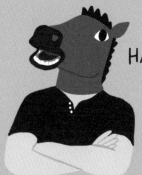

HALLOWEEN MASK

Clearly you're someone who savors the holidays all year round...

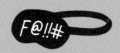

RUDE MASK

Curse words are your jam! They're so funny! They're also a warning to anyone who might disturb you and set off your hair-trigger temper!

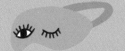

"REALISTIC" EYE MASK

Whether it's googly eyes, a humanoid face, or a reptile with one eye open, well, it's creepy. Stop that.

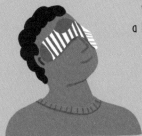

SOCKS

It's unclear whether you are wearing socks over your eyes on purpose or if a rogue child put them there because you fell asleep during playtime. Get some rest, honey.

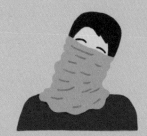

NECK WARMER PULLED OVER YOUR FACE

You're industrious and resourceful, and you can still see some light, but at least you don't have to make eye contact with anyone.

HAMMERHEAD PILLOW

You're desperately hoping to stick your head in the sand for several years. Good luck being respected by anyone who sees you wearing this pillowy tree stump.

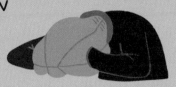

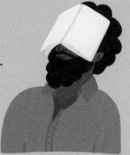

COOLING GEL MASK

Wellness is your middle name. Are you a) having night sweats or b) wearing a faceberg because you heard it might un-puff your under-eye circles?

A CAT

Can you breathe under there? What's that? You're allergic to cats?

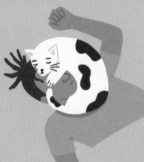

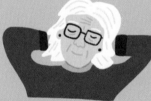

A BOOK

Congratulations— you are your own bookmark.

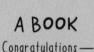

NO MASK

You're either a deep sleeper or afraid of being attacked during your nap.

BRA FOR YOUR FACE

This expensive mask is contoured to fit in your tired, sunken eye sockets.

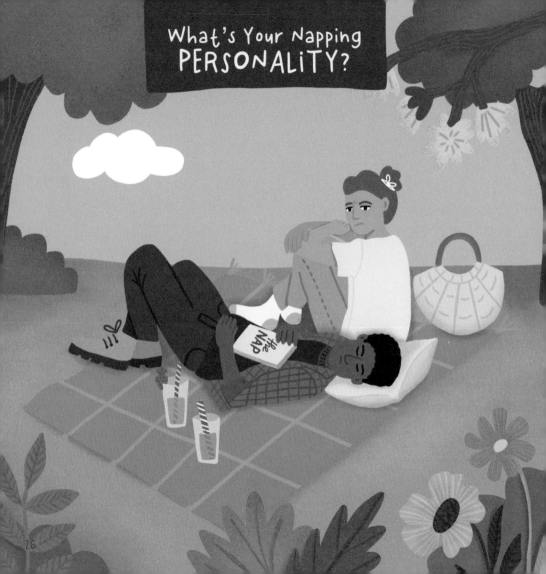

THE NEVER NAPPER

Many failed naps are the bane of this individual's existence.
A common scenario: Two subjects are observed after a leisurely
weekend brunch, which has left them full and drowsy as they
stroll through a neighborhood park. They unfurl a blanket in a sunny
spot and settle themselves in. A yawn may present itself. Upon
repose, one individual is dipatched into slumber; the other, despite
heavy eyelids and deep tiredness, experiences a ping—pong match
of the brain. With time, acceptance is possible, although some
Never Nappers forever remain deeply envious, sometimes to the
point of rage, of other people's ability to nap.

POLYMATHS* WITH POLYPHASIC** PREFERENCES

Both Leonardo da Vinci and Nikola Tesla took six 20-minute naps
spread evenly throughout the day
(a cycle of sleeping known as the Uberman cycle).

*polymath: a person whose knowledge is vast, across many subjects

**polyphasic: having two or more phases: in sleep terms it means that
you take multiple naps per day instead of one long overnight sleep

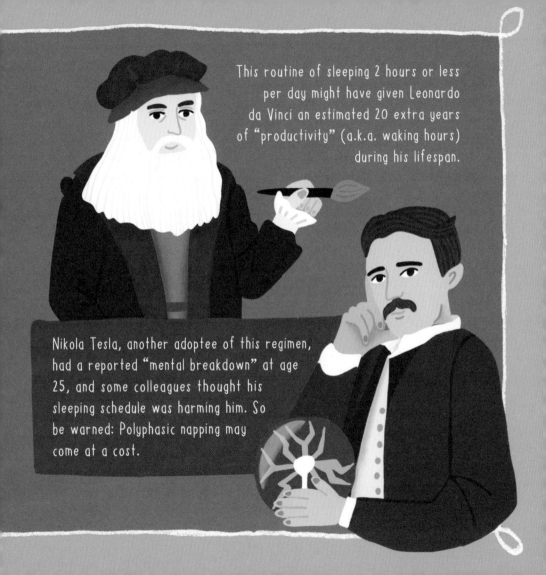

This routine of sleeping 2 hours or less per day might have given Leonardo da Vinci an estimated 20 extra years of "productivity" (a.k.a. waking hours) during his lifespan.

Nikola Tesla, another adoptee of this regimen, had a reported "mental breakdown" at age 25, and some colleagues thought his sleeping schedule was harming him. So be warned: Polyphasic napping may come at a cost.

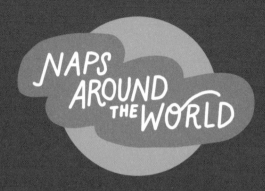

TAASEELA

The Arabic word for a midday nap in Egypt.
A two-hour afternoon nap is usually followed by a
six-hour evening sleep.

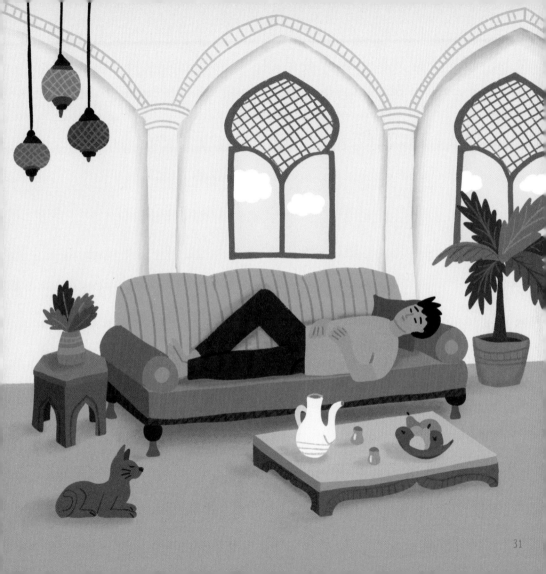

DISCO NAP

restorative pregame sleep taken before going out to a club or to a party for the evening

TIME: 30 to 90 minutes

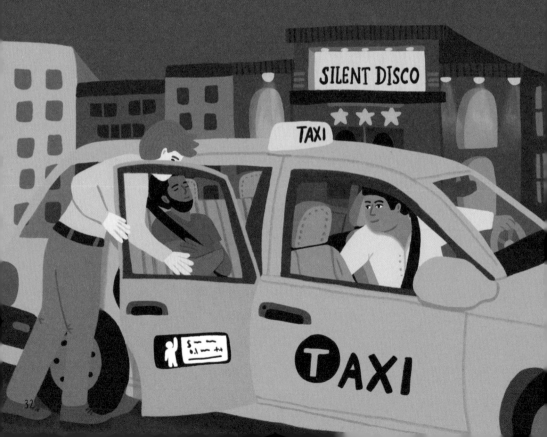

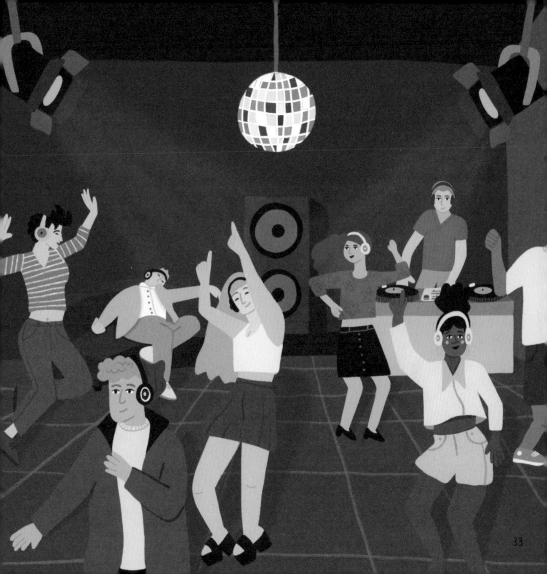

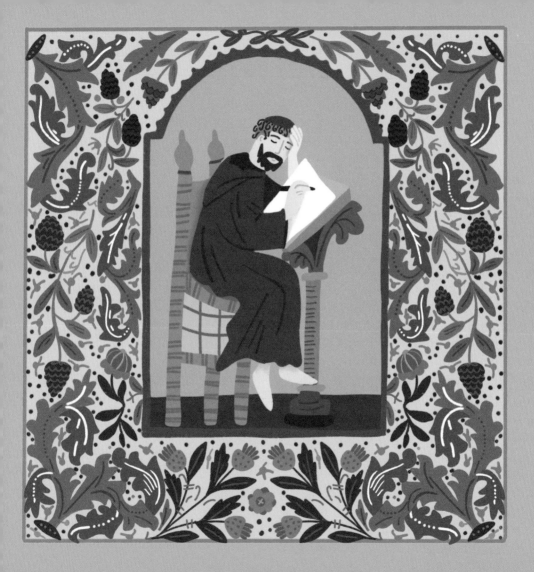

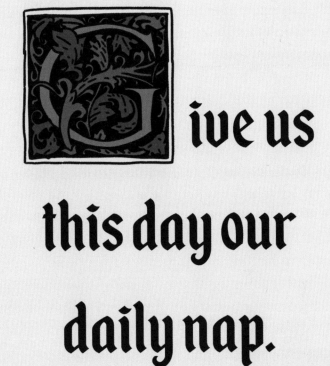

Give us
this day our
daily nap.

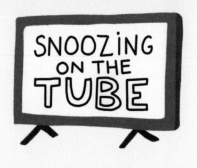

SNOOZING ON THE TUBE

TV AND NAPS JUST GO TOGETHER! HERE ARE A FEW MOMENTS WHEN THE NAP MADE TELEVISION HISTORY.

FRIENDS

In "The One with the Nap Partners," Joey and Ross accidentally take a nap together when they both fall asleep on the couch. They are very alarmed when they wake up snuggled next to each other, but they later admit that they just had the best nap of their lives.

SEINFELD

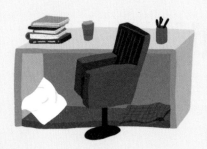

George has a bed built under his desk for naps at work—he has a glass window in his office and doesn't want to be seen snoozing. He gets an alarm clock shelf and blanket drawer constructed with the bed. The desk eventually gets dismantled after a series of haphazard events involving George Steinbrenner (his boss, the owner of the Yankees) and a bomb squad.

THE OFFICE

Stanley Hudson is a nap champion. He sometimes falls so deeply asleep in various situations that he has become a bit of a meme for zonking out at work. He wears a mask one Halloween so that he can nap at his desk without being noticed. Only once, when he drinks a massive amount of espresso from the new office machine, does he stay awake past 2 p.m.

30 ROCK

When Liz Lemon asks Jack Donaghy how he sleeps at night, he informs her that... he doesn't! Apparently Jack takes "thousands of micro naps" during the day. He takes one right in front of her and it lasts all of three seconds.

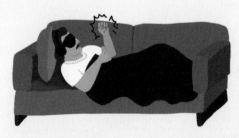

PARKS AND RECREATION

Ron Swanson takes a nap because he's been given the 4 a.m. to 6 a.m. time slot of a telethon that Leslie Knope has volunteered for. When Leslie tries to wake him to get him to help her, she finds him on a couch, wearing a sleep mask and violently punching the air. Of course, Ron explains that he has a sleep fighting disorder. When Leslie says that the problem must be terrible, Ron says, "Only when I'm losing."

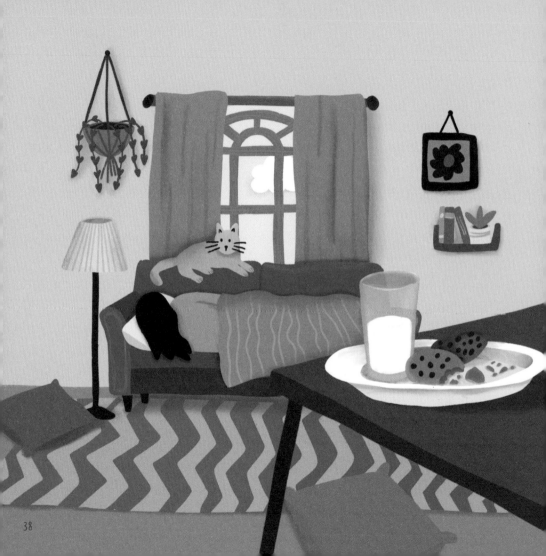

"Think what a better world it would be if we all, the whole world, had cookies and milk about three o'clock every afternoon and then lay down on our blankets for a nap."

—Barbara Jordan, a disabled lawyer, civil rights activist, and LGBTQ+ icon, who was the first Black woman elected to the Texas State Senate and the first Black Texan in Congress

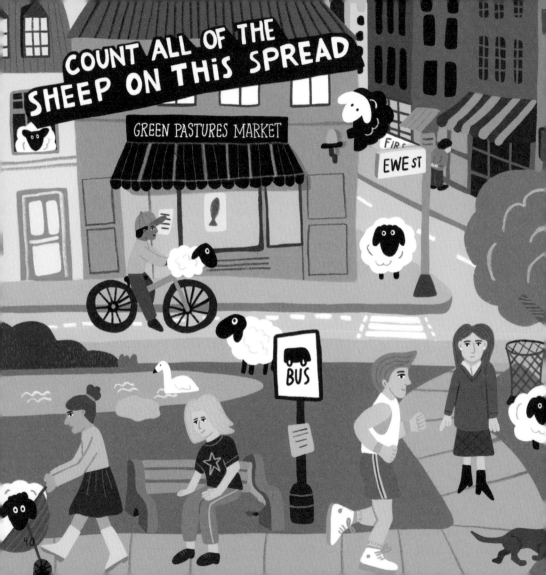

COUNT ALL OF THE
SHEEP ON THIS SPREAD

GREEN PASTURES MARKET

FIRS
EWE ST

BUS

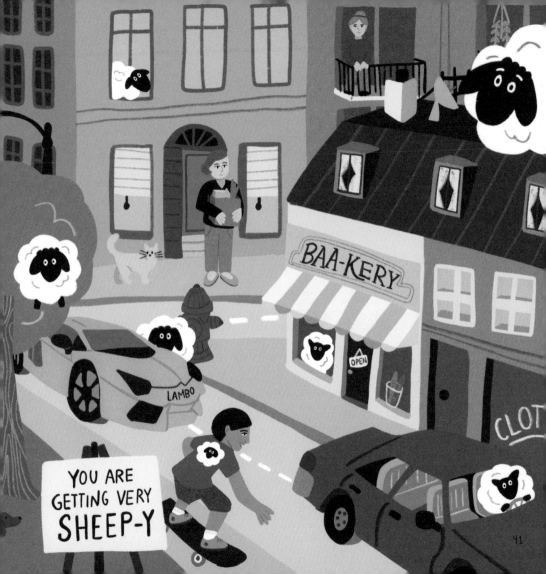

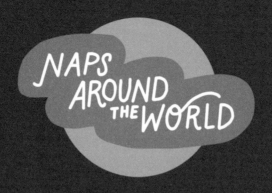

FRILUFTSLIV

"Outdoor living" in Norwegian. Babies in Scandinavia enjoy short snoozes outside in chilly temperatures—it's thought to help their sleep schedule and overall health.

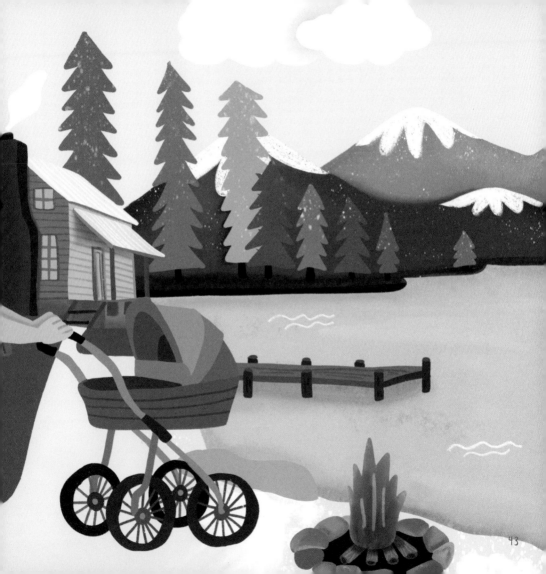

NOT JUST FOR CATS

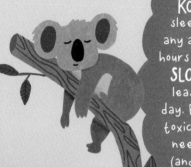

KOALAS seem to sleep the most of any animal—up to 22 hours a day. Sleepy **SLOTHS** slumber at least 15 hours per day. Both eat mostly toxic leaves so they need lots of rest (and don't take in many calories).

You may have heard of a **CAT** nap... but are cats the only animals that take a midday slumber? No! Lots of creatures snooze during the day.

DOGS need naps! Puppies need to rest up to 18 hours per day; adult dogs closer to 14.

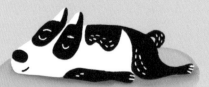

SNAKES nap with both eyes open. (They have no eyelids.)

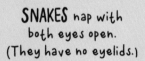

Zzz...

BATS can lock their feet into place to nap upside down.

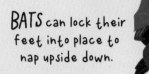

A study of the **GREAT FRIGATEBIRD** found that it sleeps in flight—coasting on the breeze in updrafts of air.

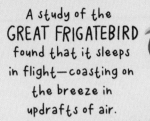

OTTERS take naps in a "raft" with other floating otters—sometimes they hold hands to sleep.

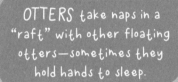

DOLPHINS and **WHALES** sleep while they swim and can remain partially awake (known as unihemispheric sleep—one side of the brain remains awake while the other sleeps), swimming slowly next to another or, for whales, resting vertically in the water.

45

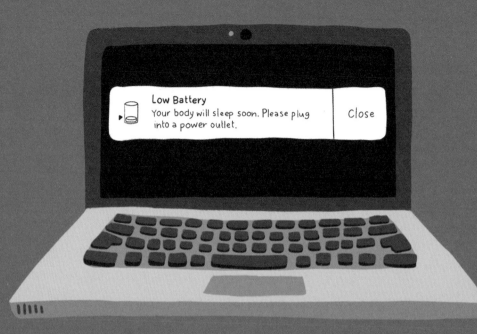

POWER NAP

a short sleep taken during the day to boost vitality

TIME: 20 minutes

Cornell University social psychologist James B. Maas coined this term; 20 minutes of nap time is enough to increase alertness and motor skills upon waking.

NAPPiNG POWER POSES

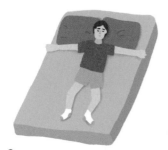

Super-Starfish

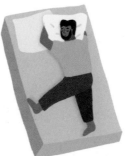

Roundhouse Kick

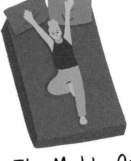

The Mighty Oak

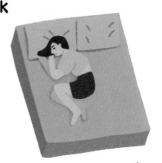

El Capitan

Cannonball

Being unconscious for 30 to 60 minutes of the workday gets you to 5 p.m. even faster.

It's a valid excuse for those who never make their beds in the morning. Why make it look pretty when you're about to get back in and mess it up?

Pants are optional.

All the best people take naps.

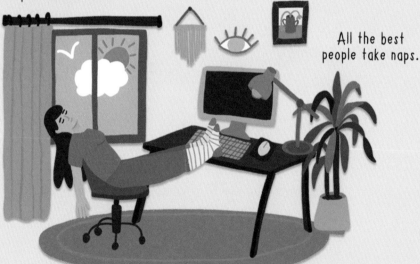

If you wake up sweaty, you can count your nap as catching up on sleep AND as a workout.

It's hard to be stressed during a nap.

Your brain works through your memories and emotions while you nap and wakes up rebooted.

...AND CONS OF NAPPING

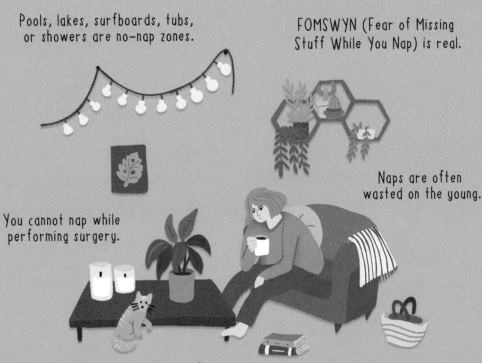

Pools, lakes, surfboards, tubs, or showers are no-nap zones.

FOMSWYN (Fear of Missing Stuff While You Nap) is real.

Naps are often wasted on the young.

You cannot nap while performing surgery.

If your employer is advocating for naps at work, beware...they might be tempting you into a culture of longer working hours and being on call 24/7.

Naps are often unsuccessful on roller-coaster rides.

49

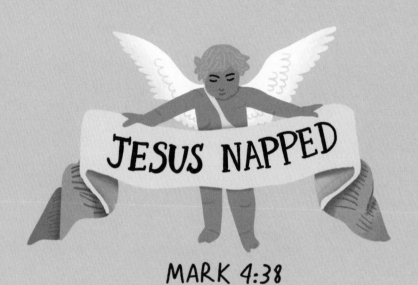

JESUS NAPPED

MARK 4:38

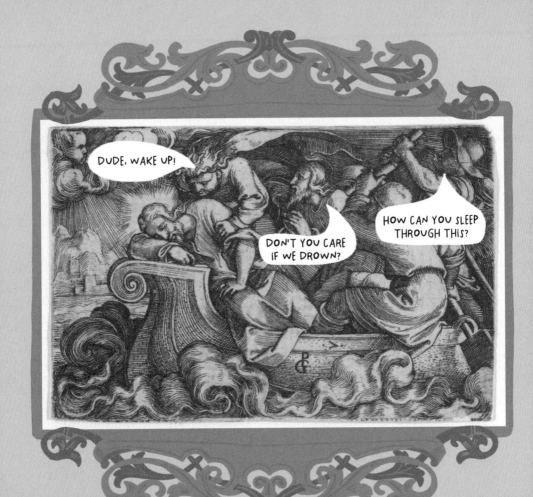

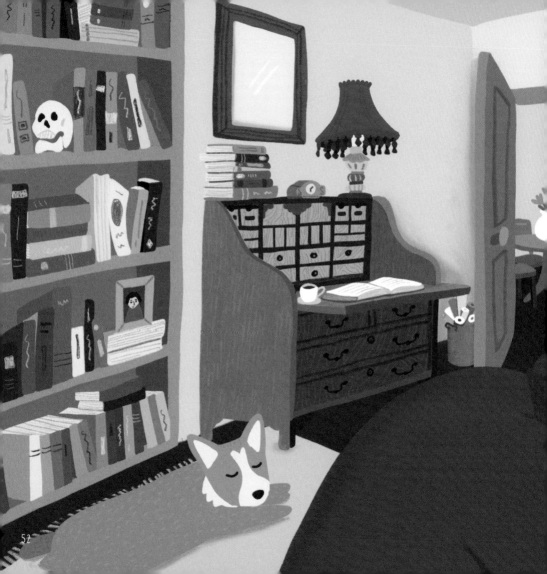

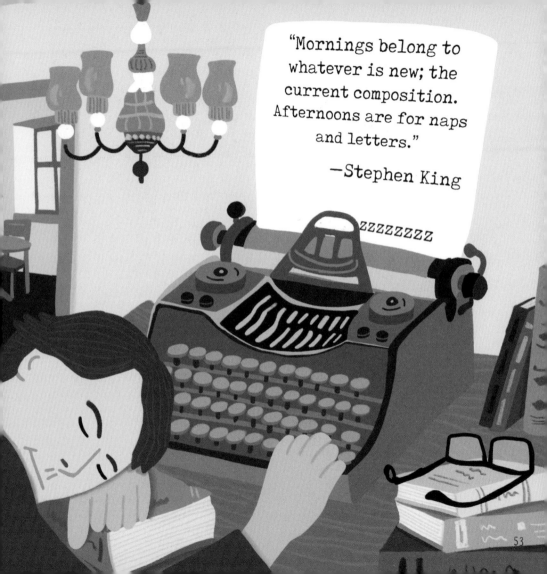

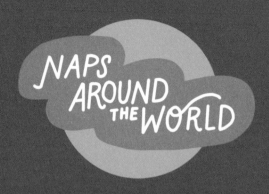

NAPS AROUND THE WORLD

VAMKUKSHI

An Ayurvedic (Hindu medicine) technique of lying down on the left side of the body after a meal to promote digestion.

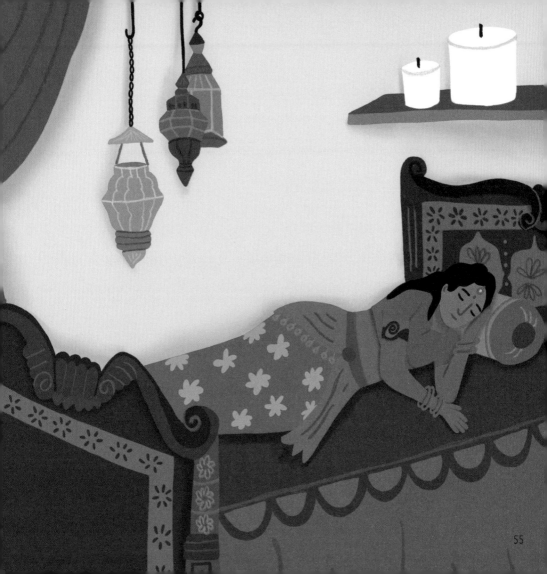

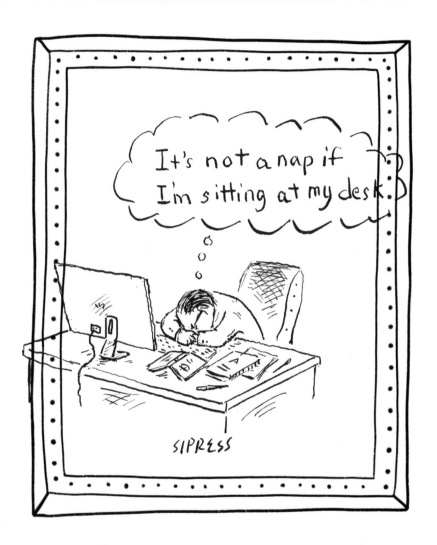

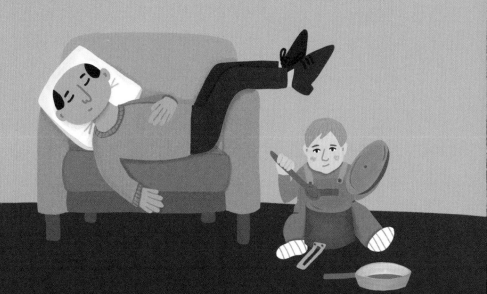

THE ONE WHO NAPS LiKE THE DEAD

Often observed while very deep in sleep, perhaps in the middle of a busy household. This napper cannot be roused by excessively close lawn mowing, a cacophony of banging pots and pans, cries of a chorus of toddlers, a phone ringing at full volume, golf ball–sized hail on a tin roof, or the screams of an intruding hyena. Check in to see if they are late for a meeting or if their breathing has dipped below the desired threshold for life. Techniques for awakening them vary; some success has been shown after yelling, "The dog is vomiting on your favorite sweatshirt!"

HOW TO TAKE A SECRET NAP

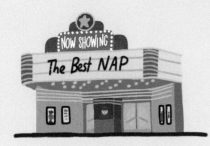

Go to a movie theater by yourself and sit in the back. Make sure you read the synopsis of what happened during the parts of the movie you slept through.

Visit a public pool and take over a lounge chair (best in hot weather; don't forget sunscreen).

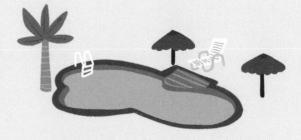

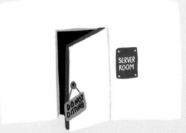

Build a hideaway in an inconspicuous area of your office. (Who goes in that server room, anyway?)

Bring your hammock to the park during a lunch break.

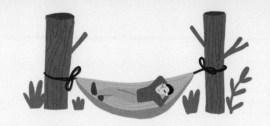

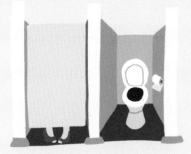

Take over a bathroom stall (ew).

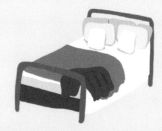

At a friend's dinner party, pretend to go to the bathroom, locate a comfy-looking bed, and dive in.

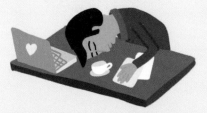

Just put your head on your desk and hope no one notices.

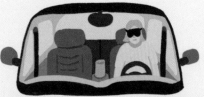

Drive your car to a secure location, roll back your seat, apply eye mask, and voilà.

SLEEP INERTIA

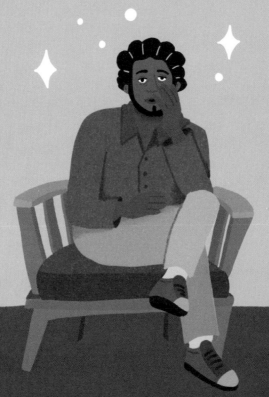

feeling of grogginess, slowness, brain fog, or disorientation after
waking up, particularly from a nap; the deep desire to return to sleep

POTENTIAL CAUSES:

- Waking up during slow-wave (non-REM) sleep
- High levels of adenosine, a neurotransmitter that increases sleep drive
- General sleep deprivation
- Naps longer than 30 minutes

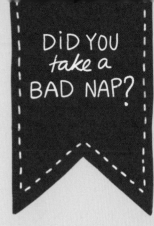

DID YOU *take a* BAD NAP?

POTENTIAL REMEDIES:

- Choose a certain time of day, ideally 8 hours after you wake up and 8 hours before you go to bed.

- Set an alarm: 20- to 30-minute naps will give you the benefits of alertness but won't take you into deep sleep (so they're easier to wake from).

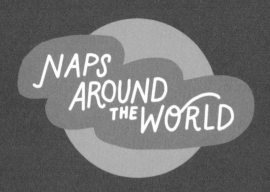

NAPS AROUND THE WORLD

RIPOSO

Italian for "afternoon nap"—much like a siesta, it takes place between 2 p.m. and 4 p.m.

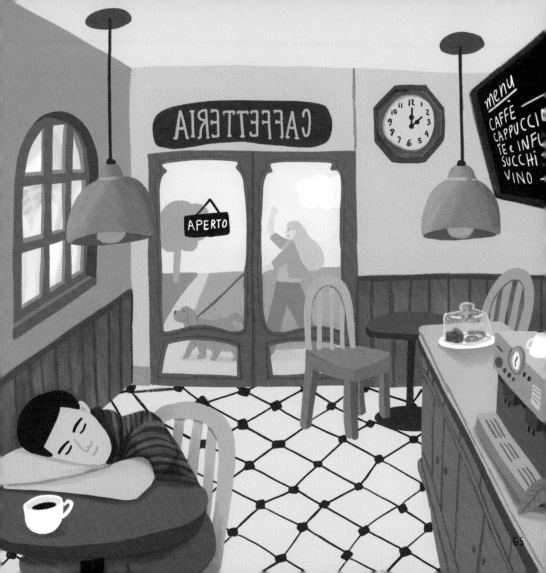

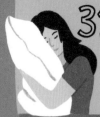

31% of AMERICANS (who work from home) nap during the workday

NAPPING BY THE NUMBERS

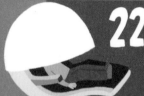

22% of AMERICANS (with in-office jobs) nap during the workday

6% of U.S. employers provide nap rooms

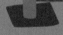

85% of MAMMALS are polyphasic

(see page 28)

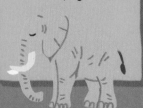

$411 billion per year: amount of MONEY estimated to be lost from the U.S. economy due to sleep deprivation

(equivalent of 1.2 million workdays)

20% increase in BRAIN function for people who study something, nap for 90 minutes, and then take a test

8% STOMACH SLEEPERS

54% SIDE SLEEPERS

38% BACK SLEEPERS

PEOPLE WHO NAP HAVE...

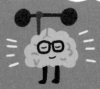

- improved memory and performance
- lower frustration
- boosted creativity
- reduced stress
- higher energy levels

BETWEEN THE HOURS OF 2 P.M. AND 4 P.M., HUMANS ARE MORE LIKELY TO:

- get in a traffic accident
- miss seeing a polyp on a colonoscopy
- be unethical or dishonest
- perform worse on a test
- issue an unfavorable ruling for a prisoner

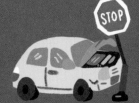

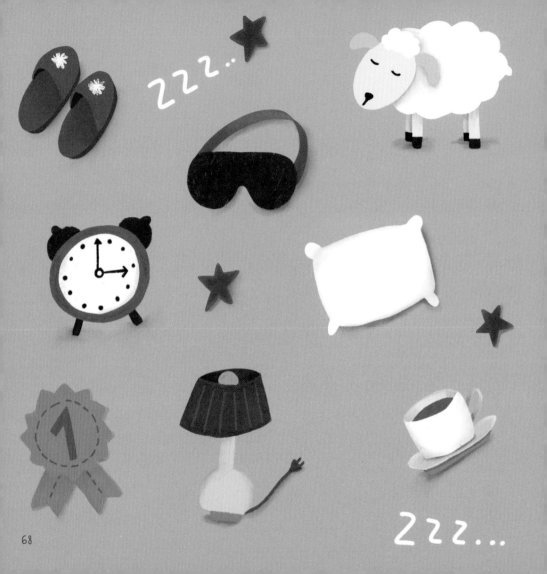

zzz..

zzz...

Napping is my Favorite Sport

CAT NAP

a light daytime sleep

TIME: 15—20 minutes

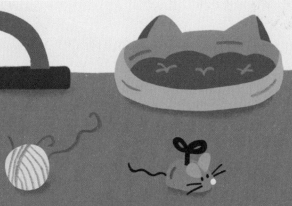

FELiNE PURRFECT AFTER A NAP

- average length of nap for a cat: 78 minutes
- cat's preferred waking time: dawn or dusk
- average total time cats spend napping per day: 12–18 hours

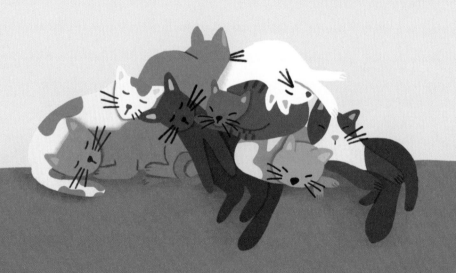

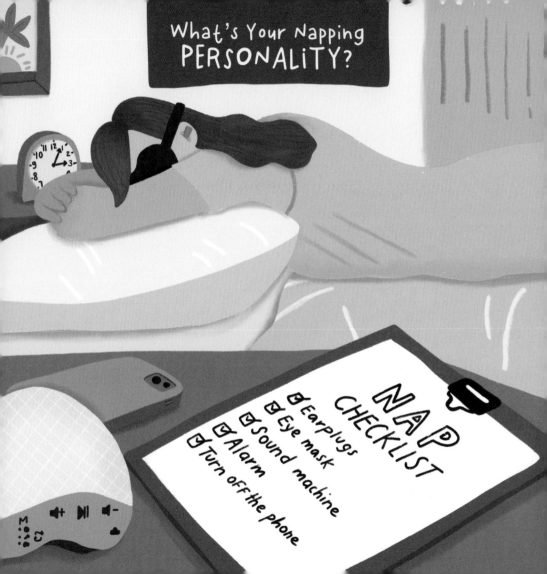

THE REGIMENTED NAPPER

Just as the sun sets in the west at a predictable time,
so does this napper turn to their sacred sleep spot at a
precise moment in the day. Preparations are made, including
application of earplugs and scented eye mask, initiating a
sound machine, drawing blackout curtains, and situating the
pillow just so, until ritual gives way to a precise amount
of slumber, carefully calibrated to end at the optimum waking
moment with the jingle of an alarm or the gradual brightening
of a sunlight—mimicking lamp. A true scientific phenomenon.

GREAT NAPPERS IN HISTORY

"The most vigorous and alert condition I have ever enjoyed."

—architect and inventor
BUCKMINSTER FULLER on his "Dymaxion" sleep schedule, which involved taking a 30–minute nap at the first moment he noticed fatigue, roughly every six hours, and which he followed for two years until his wife could no longer put up with it.

"May we learn to honor the hammock, the siesta, the nap and the pause in all its forms."

— **ALICE WALKER**

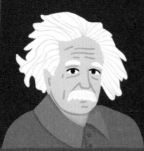

ALBERT EINSTEIN'S daily schedule while at Princeton University:

9 a.m.—10 a.m.: breakfast and newspapers
10:30 a.m.: walk to the office
11 a.m.—1 p.m.: work, then walk home
1:30 p.m.: lunch, nap, cup of tea
Afternoon: more work, correspondence
6:30 p.m.: dinner, followed by more work

"Mediterranean Yoga": **JOAN MIRÓ'S** term for a five-minute nap taken after lunch.

British PM **MARGARET THATCHER** had a reputation for sleeping only four hours a night. That sleep deficit must have caught up with her on daily drives. Her official limousine was modified with a custom headrest so that she wouldn't injure her neck during one of her frequent car naps.

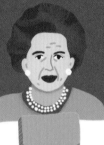

A day in the life of architect

FRANK LLOYD WRIGHT

4 a.m.–7 a.m.: drafting work
7 a.m.: first nap
Morning activities: meetings, phone calls, work with colleagues and students
At some point in the afternoon: another nap, taken on a hard surface to prevent oversleeping
4 p.m.: teatime
7:30 p.m.: dinner

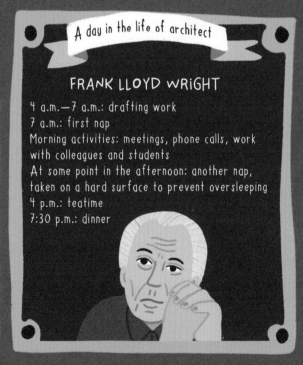

"WHAT DAY IS IT?"

Adenosine, a neurotransmitter, builds up in the human brain during waking hours and makes your body feel tired and sleepy. During sleep, adenosine levels fall. However, if your brain can't clear all of it (perhaps due to a shorter sleep, like a nap), adenosine may linger as you wake and cause confusion and grogginess.

A little bit of waking confusion can be called sleep inertia (see page 62), but more severe cases are known as "sleep drunkenness" or "confusional arousals." Sleep drunkenness can be dangerous if you wake up in a perilous situation, such as on a ship deck, and can last as long as four hours. Forgetfulness, slowness, lack of coordination, and slurred speech are all symptoms.

"I usually take a two-hour nap from one to four."

—YOGI BERRA

ANIMALS THAT AUDITIONED FOR THE JOB OF SLEEP AIDE

(...and ultimately lost to sheep)

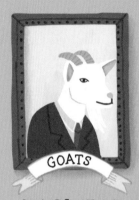

GOATS

CONSIDERATIONS:
enjoy sleep,
devil-may-care attitude

REJECTED FOR:
head-butting people awake

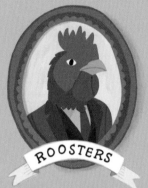

ROOSTERS

CONSIDERATIONS:
punctual

REJECTED FOR:
irritating wakefulness,
unable to silence alarm

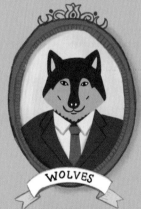

WOLVES

CONSIDERATIONS:
vigilant watch-keepers, inspire feelings of safety

REJECTED FOR:
too many "loners," too sneaky in packs

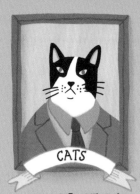

CATS

CONSIDERATIONS:
some naps were named for them

REJECTED FOR:
being cats

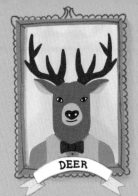

DEER

CONSIDERATIONS:
gentle, shy presence may induce naps

REJECTED FOR:
all asleep during nap time, unable
to be counted

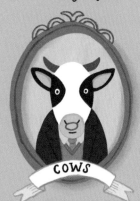

COWS

CONSIDERATIONS:
herd mentality

REJECTED FOR:
loud moo-ing not conducive to rest

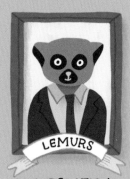

LEMURS

CONSIDERATIONS:
good in groups, gregarious

REJECTED FOR:
settling disputes with
"stink fighting"

79

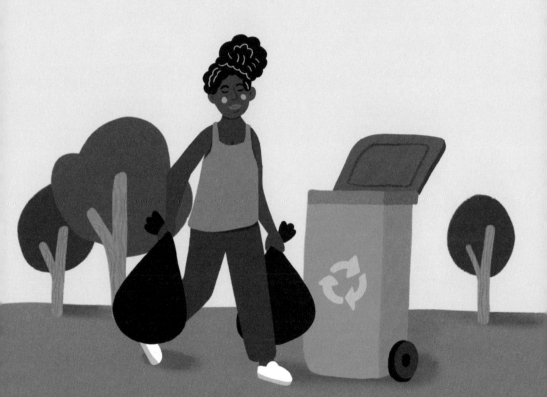

THE NAP-WALKER

Wondering where the cheese crackers went? Check for an amnesiac lumbering toward the pantry during the afternoon hours. Much like their nocturnal counterparts, this napper, though a rare specimen, is blissfully unaware of their activities —after all, they are asleep—but as daytime sleepwalkers, their somnambulism becomes more socially acceptable.
Hide the car keys.

RECOVERY NAP

daytime snooze to recoup sleep for
anyone who doesn't get enough at night

TIME: less than 30 minutes

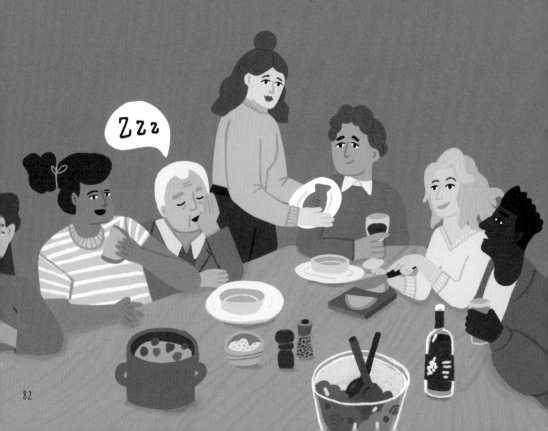

BE KIND TO YOUR BODY ... ERASE YOUR SLEEP DEFICIT!

Sleep debt is cumulative and hard to catch up on ... but it helps to nap!
When you're sleep deprived, excess cortisol (the "stress" hormone) floods
your brain. When levels of cortisol are too high, it can be harmful
to all of the systems in your body!

Most commonly, sleep deficits add up because of:

–working too late

–commuting

–socializing

–watching TV

–revenge bedtime procrastination
(a phenomenon in which a person, who has little time
for themselves during the day, stays awake too late in an
effort to exert some kind of control over their schedule)

HOW LONG SHOULD I NAP?

You may reach hypnagogic sleep and be inspired by wakeful dreams, losing consciousness very briefly.

The perfect amount of nap time, according to a NASA study, which showed that nappers were 50 percent more alert and 34 percent better at certain tasks than non-nappers.

5 MINUTES

25.8 MINUTES

20 MINUTES

Mostly stage 2 sleep — you'll be more rested when you wake up.

30 MINUTES

The exact time it will take for caffeine to kick in as you nap.

WHAT TIME OF DAY IS IT?

morning naps = more REM sleep
midday naps = both REM and deep sleep
evening naps = more deep sleep

You'll be fresh — this length of nap improves performance 34 percent and improves alertness 100%.

40 MINUTES

You will complete an entire sleep cycle, including REM sleep.

90 TO 120 MINUTES

60 MINUTES

A snooze for an hour boosts alertness for 10 hours, has the same effect on memory as a night of sleep, and helps regulate emotions.

8 HOURS

Hey...that's not a nap!

THE SLEEP CYCLE

falling asleep, 1 to 5 minutes

STAGE 1

STAGE 2

light sleep, first cycle lasts 25 minutes, memory consolidation is happening

REM (rapid eye movement) sleep, first cycle occurs 90 minutes after falling asleep, the brain is dreaming and active

STAGE 4

STAGE 3

the deepest stage of sleep, cycle starts about 45 minutes into sleep, the body is restoring and repairing itself

85

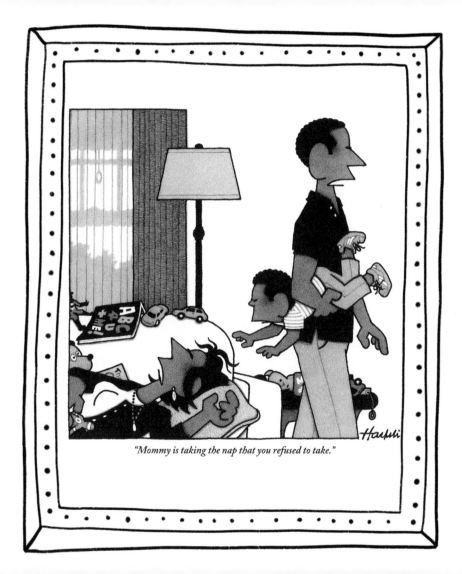

"Mommy is taking the nap that you refused to take."

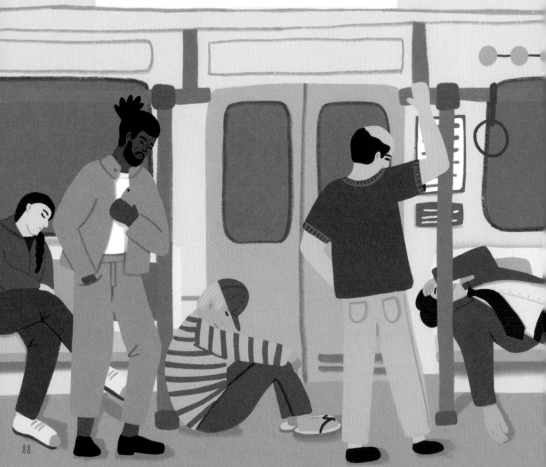

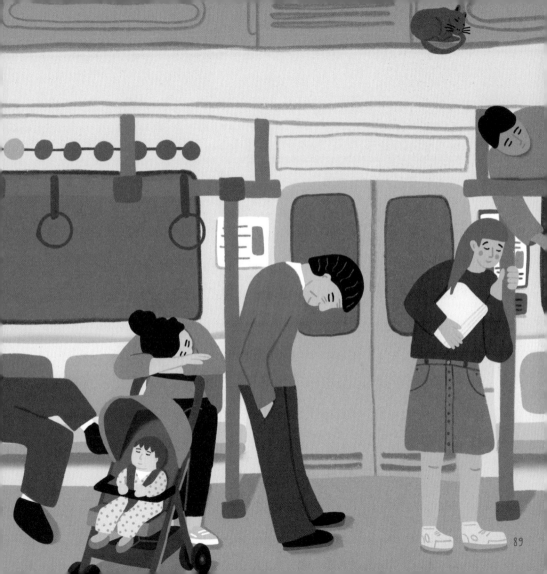

89

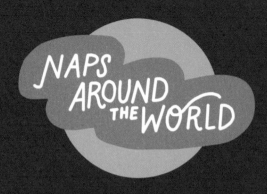

NAPS AROUND THE WORLD

SiESTA

Whether in Spain or Latin America, a siesta is a nap taken just after lunch, typically between 2 p.m. and 5 p.m.

The word comes from the Latin word *sexta* for "sixth," because ancient Romans paused their activities during the sixth hour of the day to rest.

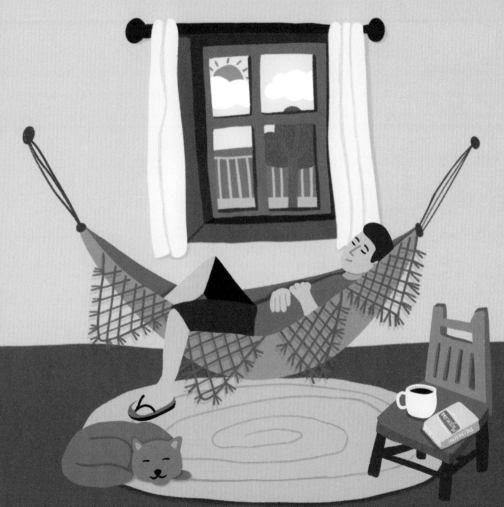

PROPHYLACTIC NAP

the nap of someone about to stay awake for a long time*

TIME: 90 minutes

*Perhaps to pull an all-nighter, work the night shift, or get up in the middle of the night to go to the airport.

NAPS ON THE NIGHT SHIFT

The American Academy of Sleep Medicine Standards of Practice Committee recommends naps for people whose working hours stretch overnight.

Whether a nap is possible during a long shift depends on the working environment. But studies have shown that napping before, during, or after a shift can help shift workers stay alert on the job and on the drive home. Napping can help combat fatigue—a common result of night shift work—and "sleep pressure," which builds up in the wee hours. Both short and long naps can increase alertness. It's not sleeping on the job when it helps you work safely and efficiently!

93

FICTIONAL
CHARACTERS
WHO TOOK SERIOUS NAPS

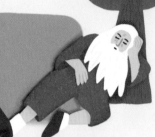

RIP VAN WINKLE

- length of nap: 20 years
- what happens when he wakes: He finds that his beard is extremely long and that he slept through the American Revolution.

GARFIELD

- frequency of naps: at least 4 per day
- cause: nap attacks
- what happens when he wakes: Time for lasagna!

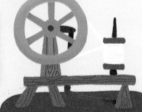

GULLIVER

- length of nap: 9 hours
- cause of nap: swimming to shore after a shipwreck
- what happens when he wakes: He finds himself tied down with stakes, with a man no more than 6 inches tall standing on him.

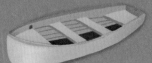

SLEEPING BEAUTY

- length of nap: 100 years
- what happens when she wakes: Her true love, a prince, is making moves on her.

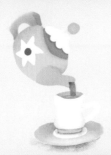

ALICE

- length of nap: 12 chapters
- what happenes when she wakes: She finds herself on a riverbank, out of the rabbit hole. Was it a dream? Was it real? Who knows...

JULIET

- length of nap: two and forty hours
- cause: Friar Laurence's vial of distilling liquor
- what happenes when she wakes: She discovers that Romeo thought she was dead, and we all know how that ended.

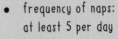

SNOOPY

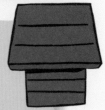

- frequency of naps: at least 5 per day
- name for a short nap: nap snack
- preferred napping place: the top of his doghouse

SNORLAX

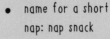

- length of nap: pretty much all day
- what will wake him from his nap: the melody of a Poké flute
- what happens when he wakes: He is very hungry!

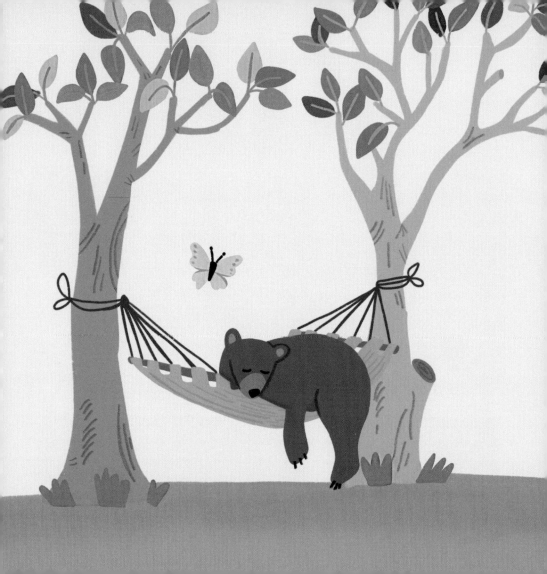

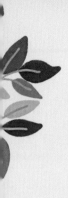
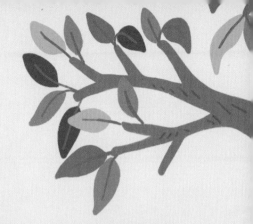

"NAPS ARE NATURE'S WAY OF REMINDING YOU THAT LIFE IS NICE—LIKE A BEAUTIFUL, SOFTLY SWINGING HAMMOCK STRUNG BETWEEN BIRTH AND INFINITY."

—PEGGY NOONAN

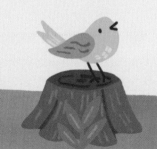

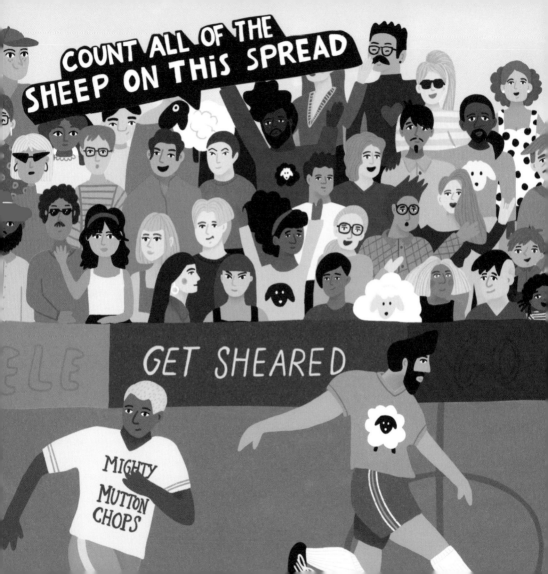

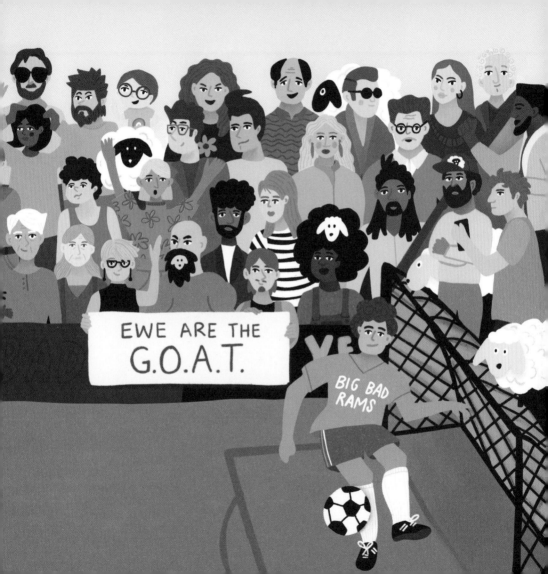

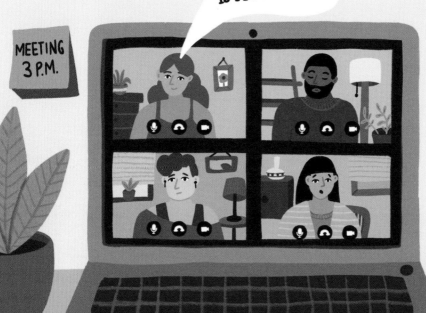

THE NAP THIEF

Can you truly be proven to nap, sweet stealer of sleep? A slumber artist and master of deception, this species of napper may not ever reveal their secrets, much less the fact that they nap at all. Attending a virtual conference? A lifelike video loop may serve as subterfuge; the nap commences. Spare 15 minutes in the car before a dentist's appointment? A nap shall be had. Waiting in line at the post office? In the middle of hot yoga class? During a house party? A thief's techniques are mysterious indeed.

"It is thou who drawest the veil of night upon the tired eyes of the day to renew its sight in a fresher gladness of awakening."

—RABINDRANATH TAGORE

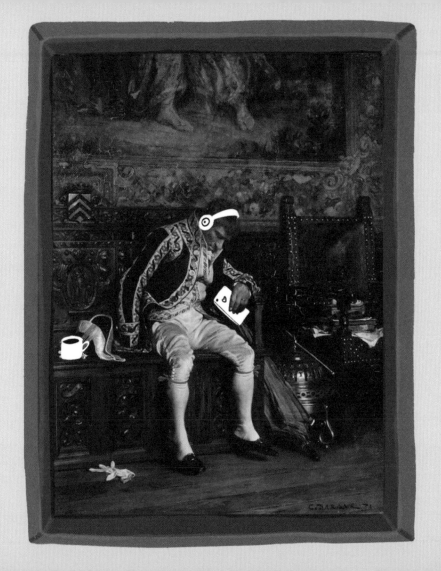

SLUMBER with a key

Artist Salvador Dalí employed a nap routine that he called "slumber with a key"—a technique that he said he learned from the Capuchin monks of Toledo, Spain.

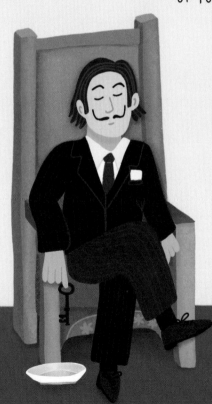

Here's Dalí's napping method:

- Place a plate or saucer on the floor.
- Sit in an armchair with your head tilted back.
- Dangle your arms down, holding a heavy key in one hand, over the saucer.
- Let yourself surrender to sleep.
- Relish the loss of consciousness that happens between letting go of the key and being jolted awake when the key hits the plate.

"I have discussed this matter at great length with scientists. Can the interval between the moment when the fingers let the key drop and the noise which it makes on the dish be considered 'sleep'? Most of them are of the opinion that true sleep occurs only five or six seconds later. Others, on the contrary, believe that this varies according to the individual."

—Salvador Dalí, in his book *50 Secrets of Magic Craftsmanship*

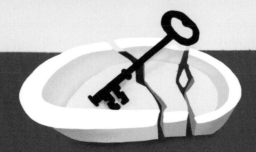

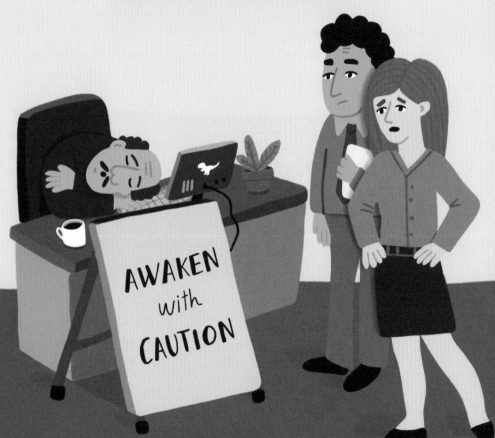

GRUMPASAURUS BRONTONAPTOR

No matter the environment or time, this napper's body cannot calibrate itself to daytime sleep, and any pleasant attitude or personality present pre-nap seems to be twisted or lost completely during the sleep cycle. This napper may have been lulled into a false sense of security by many days without a nap and the desperate scent of sleep deprivation. Despite consequences to any immediate family members, it is sometimes necessary for them to nap to remember how naps don't work for them.

(See also The Never Napper, page 27)

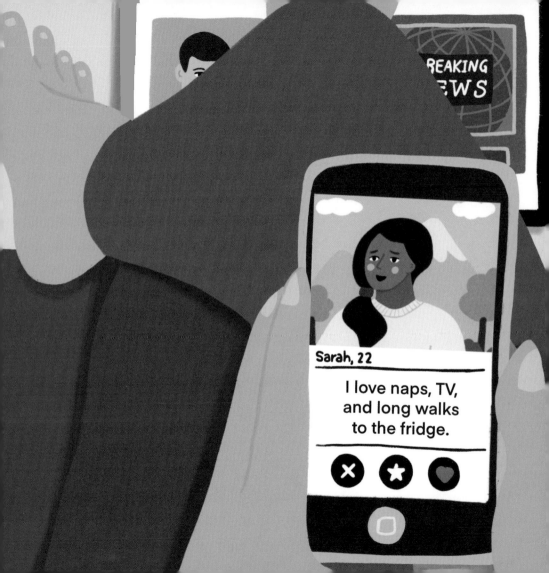

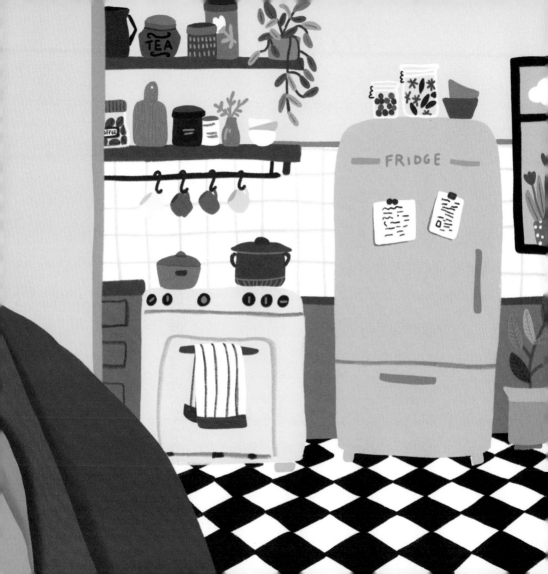

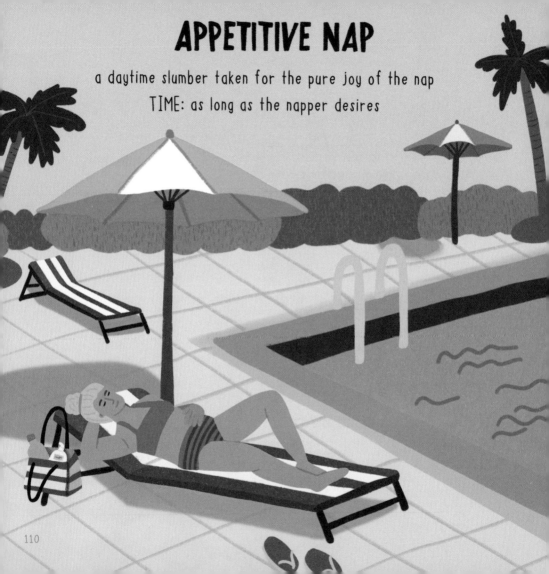

APPETITIVE NAP

a daytime slumber taken for the pure joy of the nap
TIME: as long as the napper desires

CAN NAPS HELP PREVENT BURNOUT?
YES AND NO...

Your brain needs something new and challenging to soothe burnout, not just to stop doing whatever it is that you're burned out on. A new and challenging task (that's fun for you) stimulates dopamine receptors, the reward centers of your brain, decreasing burnout better than just rest or a vacation.

However, according to Harvard researchers, even a short nap can help your brain regenerate, improving your cognitive performance and helping you feel more restored.
So, while a nap can give your brain a break, naps are probably not a long-term solution for burnout.
Keep napping for the pure love of naps!

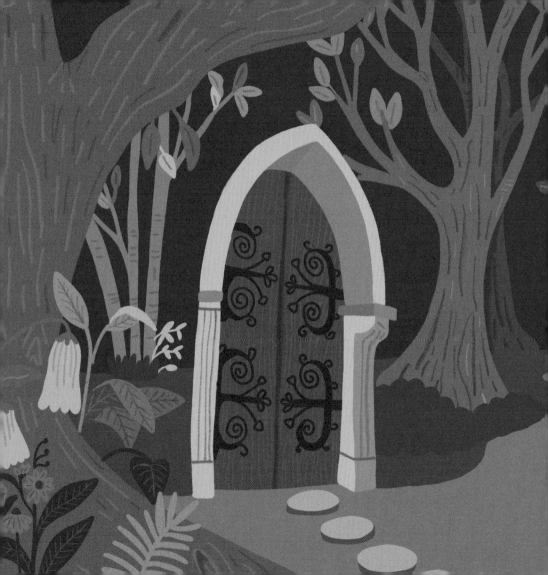

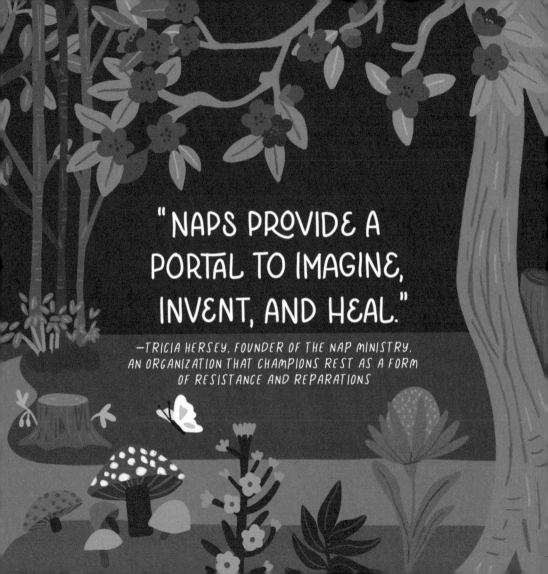

"NAPS PROVIDE A PORTAL TO IMAGINE, INVENT, AND HEAL."

—TRICIA HERSEY, FOUNDER OF THE NAP MINISTRY, AN ORGANIZATION THAT CHAMPIONS REST AS A FORM OF RESISTANCE AND REPARATIONS

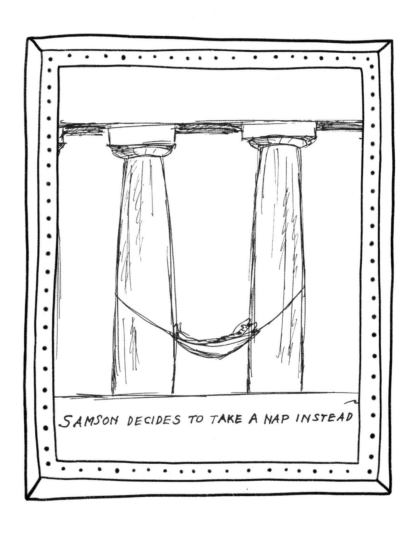

SAMSON DECIDES TO TAKE A NAP INSTEAD

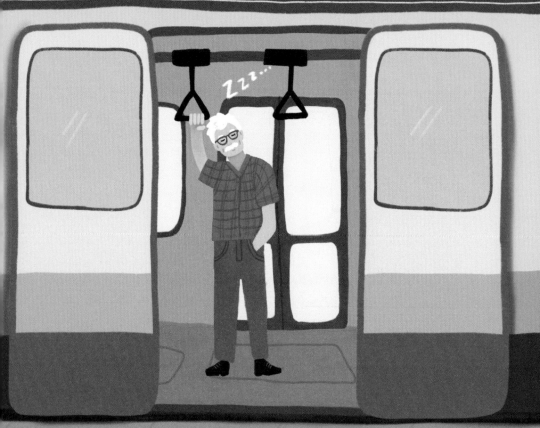

THE EQUAL NAPPORTUNIST

Whether standing, sitting, or lying flat, the Equal Napportunist can be observed drifting off into a peaceful dream state no matter the circumstances. Rattling subway cars, amphitheaters resonant with shouted Shakespeare, the sidelines of a hostile children's soccer match, a bench in the middle of a bustling shopping center, a horror show in a movie theater—nothing fazes this napper, whose public snoozing is the envy or disgust of everyone around them.

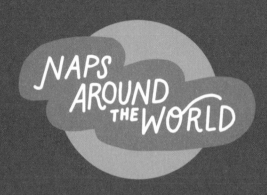

TODOET POELES

"Fear sleep"—a napping phenomenon in Balinese culture, in which the person falls instantly into a deep sleep when feeling stressed.

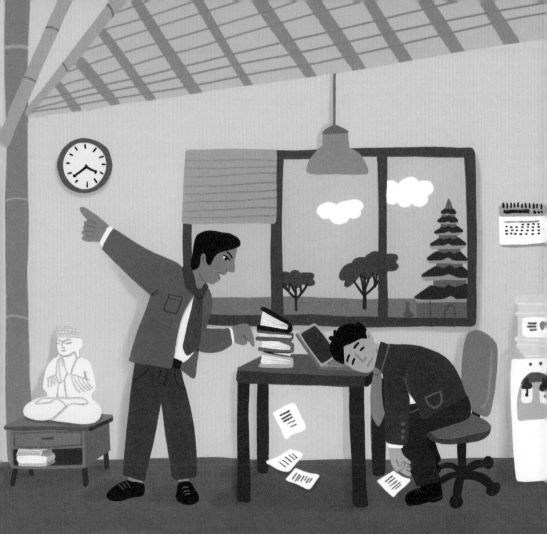

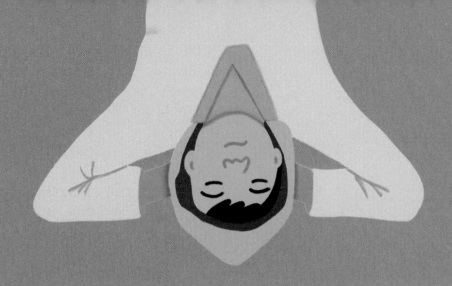

MiCRO NAP

a short burst of sleep during the day

TIME: any nap less than 20 minutes

THE "MILITARY METHOD"

Short naps sound really nice. But who wants to spend 30 minutes
trying to fall asleep, just to spend less time in slumber? Luckily, like
any elite sport, you can train for this. According to Bud Winter,
relaxation coach for the U.S. Navy Pre-Flight School, practicing
these steps will help you fall asleep anywhere, anytime:

—Relax all of the muscles of your face, including the inside of your mouth.
—Exhale, deeply relaxing your chest and upper body, muscle by muscle.
—Relax all of the muscles in your legs, telling each one to sink like a weight.
—Clear the mind for 10 seconds.
—If all else fails, repeat "don't think" for 10 seconds.

After six weeks of practicing these techniques,
most Navy pilots learned to switch on their napping mode in
120 seconds or less, regardless of the
circumstances — even
while sitting up.

COUNT ALL OF THE SHEEP ON THIS SPREAD

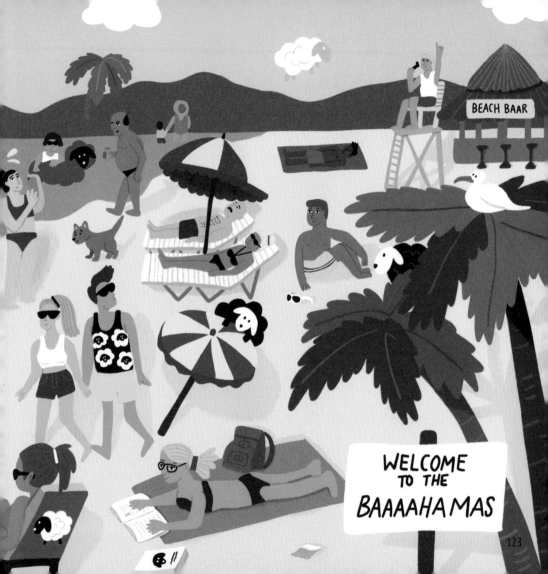

BEACH BAAR

WELCOME
TO THE
BAAAAHAMAS

123

When all else fails, take a nap.

Published by duopress, an imprint of Sourcebooks
P.O. Box 4410, Naperville, Illinois 60567-4410
(630) 961-3900
sourcebooks.com

Printed and bound in China.
RRD 10 9 8 7 6 5 4 3 2 1